HOW TO RELIEVE STRESS:

5-STEP PROGRAMS HOW TO RELIEVE STRESS AND LOSE WEIGHT FOR MEN:

CHALLENGE ONESELF - THE COURAGE TO CHANGE YOURSELF AND YOUR HABITS.

Table of Contents

Chapter 1: The Smoking Cure: How to Quit Smoking

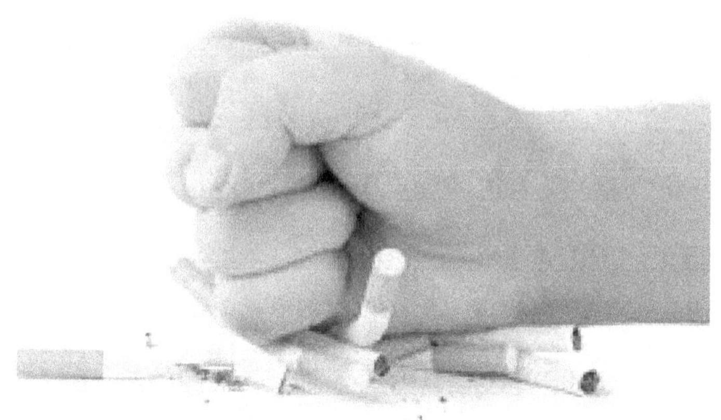

The Hazards of Smoking

Before we go into detail, remember these three important points about cigarette smoking.

- Cigarette smoking not only harms the smokers, but it also does harm to nonsmokers through second hand smoke.

- A lot of different types of cancer can be caused by cigarette smoking. This includes cancers of the larynx, esophagus, lung, kidney, throat, stomach, pancreas and cervix. Other than that, it can also cause diseases such as myeloid leukemia.

- By quitting smoking, the health risks associated with it are significantly reduced.

What Chemicals are found in tobacco smoke?

Both smokers and nonsmokers can be affected by the harmful chemicals contained in tobacco smoke. In fact, breathing just a small amount of this smoke can be very dangerous to your health. There are approximately seven thousand types of chemicals in a single cigarette stick, and of these, two hundred fifty are harmful chemicals. This includes carbon monoxide, cyanide and ammonia. Sixty-nine of these two hundred fifty chemicals can also cause cancer, and these include the following:

- Cadmium, which is a very toxic metal
- Butadiene, a hazardous type of gas
- Arsenic
- Beryllium, also a type of metal
- Benzene
- Ethylene oxide
- Chromium, which is a metallic element
- Polonium-210, a type of radioactive chemical element
- Nickel
- Vinyl chloride
- Toluene
- Benzoapyrene
- Formaldehyde

Methods for Quitting Smoking

There are many methods that one can employ to quit smoking. Using any one of these or using a combination can have differing effects from each individual so what is recommended is that you talk to an expert regarding smoking addiction and cessation and find a program that will work for you.

Nonetheless, here are some methods that you can use to quit smoking now!

1.

Cold Turkey Method

Cold turkey is a term used by people who are addicted to substances when they quit their bad habit abruptly.

This may be attributed to the fact that most addicts develop episodes of cold sweat and goose bumps during the forced withdrawal stage. This usually happens to people who take drugs like heroin or cocaine.

Unlike a heroin or cocaine addiction, a smoker does not enter into a violent withdrawal symptom stage. Although, there is an increased level of anxiety and irritability noticed in smokers who quit cold turkey. After 24 to 72 hours, this irritability and anxiety falls and there is an increased level of restlessness. Within a week, depending on the determination of the smoker to quit smoking, these symptoms are usually eradicated.

Within that 24 to 72 hour period, the body is already repairing the damage caused by smoking so quitting cold turkey does seem to be the best idea for quitting smoking.

2.

Gradual Decrease or taper Method

For those who don't choose the abrupt method, they often employ the gradual decrease method which takes a longer time. And chances are, during that period of time, the nicotine intake may increase due to several external factors like stress, anxiety and peer pressure when attending social functions.

So if it's a toss-up between cold turkey and gradual decrease of nicotine intake, stopping immediately is in your best interest. If it's any consolation; you're more likely just going to have to go through 3 days as a frazzled bird and not a cold turkey!

Although the tapering method does work for some smokers, it is still a bit risky. A good way to make this more effective is to schedule a two week tapering schedule and adhering to it.

You can also include Nicotine Replacement Therapy into the equation to help wean you off of cigarettes entirely.

3.

Nicotine Replacement Therapy

Nicotine Replacement Therapy is a method of exchanging the method by which we derive our nicotine from. Since nicotine is the active product in cigarettes that causes smoking addiction, it is only logical that there are trace amounts of nicotine in the products used for NRT. This I where Nicotine Patches, Nicotine Gums, Nicotine Lozenges and others come in.

4.

Use conventional Medicine

Although there is no "Magic pill" that can instantaneously erase smoking from our lives, there are conventional medicines that we can also use to slowly wean us off of our smoking addiction and nicotine dependency.

Two very effective conventional medicines are: Varenicline and Brupopion. Both drugs lessen the craving for nicotine and a noted side effect these two have is: it makes smoking repulsive to the smoker.

Take note that these two are prescription drugs and in no way should be used to replace smoking entirely. These two are medical aids that we can use and will work most effectively if paired with other programs like counseling and aversion therapy.

5.

Counseling

Like any form of addiction, smoking can also be cured through repeated counseling sessions. These counseling sessions may be done individually or in a group.

What counseling does is uncover the root cause of smoking and finding ways to develop step goals to getting away from the habit.

Smoking does not go away with just one counseling session though. Repeated counseling sessions helps the individual assess their progress and further motivates them to continue avoiding cigarettes. The counselor also has a way to observe the patient and find out what works and what doesn't and streamlines there program to adjust to each individual.

Other methods often used during counseling also include: hypnosis and aversion therapy.

6.

Hypnosis

Hypnosis is another method which smokers can turn to if they want to really kick the habit. Now before you think this is too New Age, hypnosis does work for some people!

But first we have to erase that initial image you have of hypnosis in your mind. This is not a stage trick you'd see in carnivals. No one can just hypnotize you and make you perform all of the silly stuff that magicians make you think they can do.

That's not how hypnosis works. Hypnosis allows you to relax and enter a trance-like state so that you can focus on a certain task or goal. In effect, it allows you to enter an altered state of mind.

During hypnosis, the patient is fully aware of what is happening in his surroundings and results vary depending on the level of cooperation between the patient and the hypnotist. The patient enters a trance like state wherein mental suggestions become easier to absorb and instill.

What takes place is basically what others would call a "mental association". What this means is that the patient goes through a series of suggestions which gives smoking a bad image in their mind. This can be through associating smoking to negative images or sensations. For example: smoking leaves a horrid taste in your mouth. This sensation is further amplified in your mind as a truly horrid taste that you begin to have an aversion to it just by thinking about it which eventually convinces you to stop smoking.

It takes several sessions for the patient to develop a strong dislike for smoking through hypnosis and for some, this might not even work. But for those whom hypnosis has worked, smoking has been completely eradicated from their bad habits.

Once again, hypnosis requires some cooperation between the patient and the hypnotist and No, the hypnotist just can't snap his fingers and your smoking addiction will disappear. You will need to work just as hard to retain those mental suggestions and practice avoidance of cigarettes at all times.

7.

Meditation

Another method that you can employ using an altered state of mind to quit smoking is through meditation.

What is meditation anyway?

Meditation is a mental conditioning that you can develop on your own after you've learned the basics. It is a great way to relax and allow your mind to go into a different form of consciousness that can help you alleviate the craving for smoking.

Everyone already knows the basics of meditation; it just takes practice to really do it. Remember when you were having a bad day and you just went out to breathe and clear your mind? That's basically how it works. Only this time, you will need a quiet place, sit down (whether on a chair or on the floor is fine) and relax. Close your eyes and try to clear your mind of any thoughts (some practitioners focus on a black wall). Breathe in deeply and slowly through your nose and exhale through your mouth. With each breath you should be able to physically feel your body relaxing more and more.

Now what this does is relieve us of anxiety which is often the main cause why we go back to smoking.

8.

Aversion Therapy

Aversion therapy is almost the same as hypnosis except it has a more physical aspect to it. What basically happens during aversion therapy is that smoking is connected to a physical stimulus that causes discomfort to the patient. This then forms a mental conditioning that is retained by most patients which has helped them quit smoking over time.

9.

Alternative measures

If there are conventional methods to address smoking addiction, there should also be alternative methods, right?

Here are some that you might want to consider:

a.

Acupuncture

Acupuncture is an ancient art and it is believed to help us stimulate our nerve centers. One of these is our pleasure center which our smoking addiction can only seem to appease. With the use of acupuncture, we can replace smoking in order to stimulate our brain to release Dopamine into our bodies.

b.

Herbal supplements

There are many herbal supplements that seem to change the taste of tobacco. This eventually helps smokers to quit smoking entirely.

c.

Magnet therapy

The use of magnets to help cure smoking addiction is still controversial but some smokers do attest to the effectiveness of magnet therapy. What happens is: two magnets are placed at opposite locations in our bodies and this seems to correct our wavelengths. You might want to give it a try to see if that works for you.

d.

Cold laser therapy

Cold laser therapy is much like acupuncture but is a more high tech form. What cold laser therapy basically does is it triggers our pleasure centers so that we get the feeling of satisfaction without the nicotine!

10.

Using sheer willpower

People can do wonders if they put their minds to it. Although this isn't something you'd normally hear, people can actually quit smoking using their will power. Just as the brain is dependent on the Dopamine released from nicotine, so can it be supplied using our brains and doing other activities that can basically keep us pre-occupied.

It takes a lot of self-control to do this but if you can manage to stay away from cigarettes for a few weeks, chances are you'll be able to stay away for a long time.

So there you have it, the methods to quitting smoking. All you have to do now is take your pick and try it for yourself. Once again, try to consult a professional who specializes in smoking addiction and cessation to help you out.

Well, you made it this far, you might as well take the time to start considering stopping your smoking addiction forever.

There are three phases involved in any form of addiction cessation: Planning phase, Implementation Phase and Continuous Program Phase. All three are essential to your success in defeating your addiction.

The Planning Phase

As with any undertaking you're about to go into, the planning phase is the most crucial part to ensure the success of your endeavor. In this case, it is ending your addiction to smoking.

Before we start:

1.

Understand that there is going to be some difficulty getting over your addiction. Although the difficulty levels vary per individual, be prepared for the worst. Just over compensate and prepare for extremely difficulty in getting over your addiction.

2.

Prioritize your program above all other tasks for the first 30 days to ensure that you will be able to quit smoking entirely.

Okay now that we have that out of the way, here are some steps you can take to prepare for the day you finally say goodbye to smoking.

1.

Mark the date on your calendar.

As with any plan, the date for implementation has to be clearly stated in order for you to make the necessary adjustments of your priorities prior to that date.

Clear your schedule and make sure that your program is the top priority.

2.

Stay away from all forms of temptations

Include this in your plan as it is important that during the 30 day program, you'll be far from temptations. If you have to take a vacation to do that, then that's what you should do. Stay away from social functions which may lead to peer pressure or even just the slightest exposure to cigarettes.

Remember: even the tiniest thing could trigger you to go back to smoking.

3.

Have the necessary medical aids

Nicotine addiction is very strong and some people may not be able to resist the temptation to go back to smoking. Have the necessary medical aids ready at hand to help you out in times of weakness.

Having a steady supply of nicotine patches and gums should help you alleviate the craving for lighting up a cigarette stick.

4.

Plan to stop completely on the implementation date.

This is pretty self-explanatory. On the first day of the 30 day program, make sure you stop completely. And don't make any excuses.

5.

Don't tell too many people about your plan to stop smoking

Although we did mention doing some counseling sessions and seeking out group therapy, don't talk to other people about your plan to quit smoking. That just might blow up in your face since you'll be raising that topic and talking about your progress when you start the 30 day program just might trigger you to go back to smoking.

Talking to your immediate family is mighty helpful though as long as they fully support your decision to quit smoking.

6.

Document your progress

As with any form of progress, documentation is crucial to help determine your strengths and areas to improve. Have a log book that you can write in ready. A calendar that you can tick off for each day that you remain smoke free will also prove very helpful to mark your progress.

You can also put a video camera and use that to document your progress.

7.

Remove all traces of smoking from your immediate surroundings

Before the start of implementation, remove everything that can serve as a trigger for you to go back to smoking. That means throwing out your ash trays, lighters and most especially your cigarettes out into the trash bin.

Now that we're done with the planning phase, it's time to get on to the implementation phase.

Always keep these things in mind:

1.

Take it one day at a time. This is probably a passage that everyone who was addicted at one point or another in their lives remembers well. The goal here is to get through the day without succumbing to the temptation of lighting up and doing the same thing tomorrow and so on and so forth.

2.

Stick to the program and stay away from all forms of temptation.

3.

It'll become easier over time. Think positive and remember all the good reasons for staying away from smoking.

4.

Say "No" and walk away. You don't need to explain yourself to anyone if someone offers you a cigarette. All you have to do is politely refuse the offer and then walk away. Don't talk about your program to stop smoking as it may lead to a lengthy discussion which could trigger the need to smoke.

5.

Keep smoking out of your mind as much as possible. Try not to have any idle time which may lead to you thinking about smoking.

6.

Don't give up when you slip up. People make mistakes all the time. Although that shouldn't be your excuse, if you do slip up and fall off the wagon, get back up as fast as you can and get right back on the program. And try your hardest not to slip up again.

7.

Don't expect the medical aids to replace the feeling of smoking. It will feel different and it will definitely taste different but nicotine gums and nicotine patches will help you by serving their main purpose which is to deliver nicotine to your system. This should help alleviate the craving for a cigarette and reduce other withdrawal symptoms and their respective effects.

8.

Like we said, it'll be difficult. Especially if we're talking about the urge to smoke. For the first week, it might seem almost unbearable to withstand but if you keep at it and restrain yourself, you'll find out that it becomes easier to resist the urge to smoke over the course of time. Just don't be discouraged.

9.

Last but not the least, most smokers who quit often gain weight. Don't worry about it. There's nothing you can do about the increase in hunger as of now. Focus all of your energy at quitting smoking and if you can put in some time for exercise, do it to keep excessive weight down.

And once you're done with the first 30 days of being completely smoke free, it's time to keep on doing what worked during your bid to end your smoking addiction.

This is the continuous program phase:

1.

The first 30 days of being smoke free was a test of your determination to get rid of your addiction. You will need to keep trying every single day not to go back to smoking.

2.

Don't fall for the "occasional cigar for special occasions" mentality. One stick and everything you've ever worked hard for can unravel.

3.

Always remain vigilant. You need to always be on guard for moments of weakness. This usually happens during times of extreme stress or extreme joy. So always be wary of what you're doing.

4.

Let's say you were able to stop completely for a couple of months, suddenly, you get that urge to smoke. These feelings do come out and it's normal. Just resist the urge for as best as you can. Usually, these urges aren't that strong anyway.

5.

Get fit and live a healthier lifestyle. You owe it to yourself and to your body for the duration of time that you were exposing yourself to health risks. Since smoking targets the heart and the lungs initially, it is in your best interest to do lots of cardiovascular activities. Walking, jogging, cycling, these are activities that can help promote good cardiovascular health.

You can also start eating healthier so that you can address the threat of cancer in your body from those years of exposure to tobacco smoke. Eating lots of vegetables with anti-oxidants is a good option and eating lots of fish and leafy greens can help bring about better hair, better skin and a better life. That's a whole lot better than what you used to have when you had that bad habit of smoking!

6.

Take up a serious hobby. One way that you can eliminate the risk of relapsing is if you take up a serious hobby and get really good at it. That should make each day that you stay nicotine free go by faster!

7.

Reward yourself with the money you've saved. Everyone needs to be rewarded for a job well done. One of the things that you can do during the implementation phase as well as the continuous program phase is to put money equivalent to what a pack of cigarettes would cost you into a savings account. That's one way that you can benefit from stopping smoking and in the end you can use that money for whatever purpose you may want it to serve.

Just don't use it to buy a pack of cigarettes though! Seriously.

In order for the program to work you have to continuously plan, implement and adhere to it. You also need to make the necessary adjustments every time the need arises.

Remember that your end goal here is to quit smoking and end your addiction. So take it one day at a time and always be vigilant!

Chapter 2: Stop Drinking Now

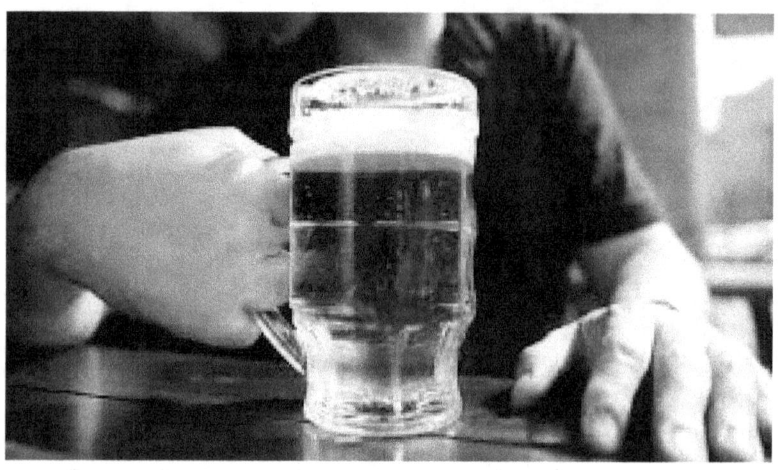

The First Step to Stop Drinking: Commit to It
One of the biggest obstacles for people who want to stop drinking is their constant denial of their problem. Most alcoholics already have people urging them to either quit drinking or to just tone it down a little. However, if the person himself does not admit that his drinking problem is an actual problem, then he wouldn't take steps to change it. This is why it is important for the person to first recognize and admit that he does have a drinking problem. Once the admission is made, he should then follow through with a commitment to stop drinking.
However, note that this process does not happen overnight. Many recovering alcoholics have had to go through a gradual process before they finally mustered up the willingness to at least try to stop drinking. Sometimes, this willingness may have been spurred by the fact that the individual has already hit rock bottom: he may have already lost important

aspects of his life. In most cases, job loss or losing one's family and social connections could be the triggering factor.

What to Do after Admitting that You are an Alcoholic

Once the alcoholic recognizes that he has to start changing his drinking patterns, he should follow this through with the following steps. These steps effectively ensure that he commits to the process and that his resolve is strengthened:

1.   Make a comparison chart of the benefits and costs of drinking and compare these with the benefits and costs of not drinking. It is best if you write these down on a diary in order to have a visual proof of the reasons why the drinking has to stop.

2.   Set the right goals. Having goals will help greatly when preparing for the arduous journey that lies ahead. When setting goals, it would also be best to be specific. For instance, instead of saying"I should stop drinking by next year", it is best to set a specific quit date.

3.   Eliminate all possible causes of temptation. This includes clearing out all the items on the bar at home, as well as every single bottle of alcohol that may be hidden in various secret hiding places. It is also best to remove all possible triggering factors that could induce the temptation to go grab a drink. These factors could be work-related or could also be something in one's personal life.

For instance, if the loss of a loved one has triggered the alcoholism, then it is best to get rid of everything that would remind of you of that person. Do not pay any regard to the sentimental value of each item, especially if that sentiment could induce you to start drinking again.

4.   Let everyone know of the intention to quit drinking. Hearing the intention said out loud could

help bolster the individual's motivation. This would also help the individual gain the support of the people around him. As every recovering alcoholic knows, emotional and social support is an invaluable aspect of the recovery process.

By announcing the intent to quit drinking, it would also be easier for the individual to set limits for the people around him. This means that they can perfectly understand in case he asks them not to drink while he's around. After all, he does have to get rid of everything that could tempt him to fall back into the old routine.

5.   Let go of the people who do not support the effort to quit. Most likely, these people could influence the individual to continue the habit. These are the very same people who wouldn't respect the boundaries that were set by the person who's trying to quit. Specifically, these people would still continue drinking in front of you even after they have been asked not to.

There are also cases wherein friends promised not to have any alcoholic drinks if the recovering alcoholic joins them on some celebration. However, as every celebration goes, alcohol is something that could never be absent. In order not to jeopardize the recovery process, it is best to get yourself out of that situation right away.

Committing to the process is easier said than done. The individual would also have to understand that alcoholism is an addiction. Just like any other addiction, quitting the habit takes a toll on the body. The process would also be fraught with so many bumps that it could sometimes be easier to just continue with the habit rather than get rid of it. This is why in most cases, the alcoholic may have already tried to quit several times in the past but failed.

This is why it is important for a recovering alcoholic to take note of his past attempts at quitting. He has to analyze the methods by which he tried to quit drinking in the past and then check why and how those methods failed. This analysis can be included on the diary so that the individual would have a visual confirmation of whether he is repeating the failed patterns or is successfully veering away from it.

Chapter 3: Good nightlife is vital

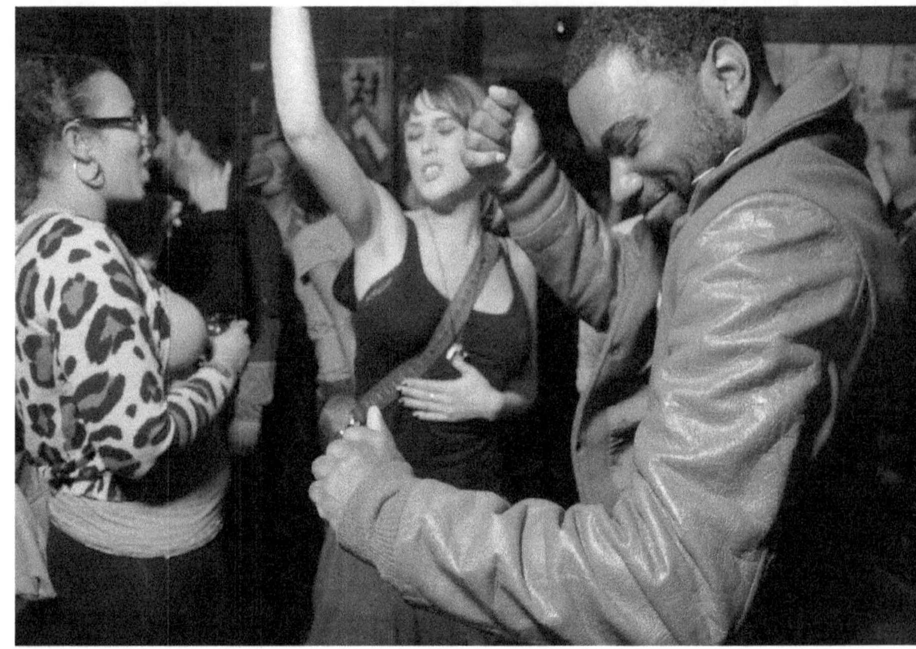

If you're reading this, you already know how nasty hangovers can be. For most of us, hangovers come with obvious symptoms. We wake up with our mouths parched, the taste of certain drinks and spirits still lingering on our tongues. Our head may be sore, or even pounding. Our limbs may hurt, our thirst is unquenchable. Sometimes we even feel queasy, with no choice but to void our stomachs. Often we have to urinate...

Put simply, hangovers ain't pretty. In their worse form, they can take a whole day to overcome. Heck, sometimes we still feel 'weird' multiple days later. In their lesser form, a quick drink of water and maybe an Advil will do the trick.

But what causes these unpleasant feelings? Is it merely dehydration? Is it the lingering effect of alcohol withdrawal on our brain and body? What happens when we overindulge and suffer the after-effects?

As it turn outs, drinking causes a whole *range* of associated symptoms. Let's quickly cover the important aspects of a hangover, so you have a better idea of what is going on in there...

Dehydration

This one is obvious. Often we talk about 'breaking the seal' when drinking, and this is because alcohol is a diuretic. It causes your body to lose fluid, meaning you lose water, electrolytes and a variety of important things your mind and body need to run effectively. Because your body withdraws water from your brain, you may feel lethargic, dizzy, or lightheaded. Not to mention, learning and memory may become significantly impaired. This happens because your brain literally shrinks when dehydrated. The cells in your brain are drying out and thus contract. Rehydrating those cells too quickly may lead to swelling of the brain, because the fluid-deprived cells soak up liquid too quickly. Cell damage and rupturing can occur.

Urination

As previously mentioned, alcohol causes you to lose fluid. This happens because alcohol prevents the release of an anti-diuretic hormone known as vasopressin. This hormone regulates our urination, but when it is suppressed, water goes straight through us to our bladders. In the end, our bodies do no sustain proper fluid retention, and important electrolytes are lost.

Glutamine Flux

As you probably know, alcohol is categorized a depressant. Because of this, it naturally suppresses the release of stimulants in your body. One such stimulant is glutamine. When glutamine is inhibited, we become drowsy and may fall asleep—or pass out—more easily. Although a lot of people may enjoy small amounts of alcohol to fall asleep quicker, there is a catch. Once drinking has ceased, the body naturally returns your levels to normal. This means that your body goes into overdrive to increase glutamine levels. Again, because glutamine is a stimulant, it will likely disrupt your sleep. This is why you may suffer from lack of quality sleep, or wake up continuously after consuming alcohol. This rebound in glutamine has been linked to lethargy, restlessness and hypertension during the hangover phase.

Circulatory Changes

Speaking of hypertension, alcohol has another powerful effect on your blood vessels. The reason we often get headaches is because our blood vessels will expand. Alcohol also effects our blood sugar levels, typically causing them to drop. This leads to hangover symptoms such as fatigue, mood changes, and seizures. Alcoholics will often experience 'the shakes' as a result of this effect. Alcohol can also lead to increased stomach acid, which causes the well-known symptoms of nausea, stomach pain and vomiting.

Increased Acetaldehyde

Never heard of this? Well, you're not alone. Acetaldehyde is a byproduct created by your liver when processing alcohol. Incredibly, this byproduct is up to **30 times** more toxic than actual alcohol. Fortunately, our body has a natural defense mechanism for this—but even that mechanism can be disrupted by enough alcohol. Women have less of the necessary enzymes and antioxidants to break down acetaldehyde, which is why they have a more severe reaction when drinking the same amount as a similarly sized man.

The Congener Effect

These unfriendly little ingredients are the reason that some people claim to get worse hangovers from certain liquors. The reason for this is that the processes of fermentation and distillation lead to byproducts. These byproducts are congeners, and these congeners are more prevalent in darker liquors like whiskey, red wine, and brandy. Clear liquors like vodka and gin have lower levels, and are believed to have less negative effects on one's hangover.

Inflammation

A final area of hangover effect is that of inflammation. Chronic inflammation has been linked to a variety of ailments, including diseases such as heart disease and cancer. Hangovers typically involve a level of immune system response. In this response, the system fights off the toxins in a manner that induces reduced appetite, concentration problems, and issues with storing, consolidating and retrieving memories.

So there you have it, some of the main biological processes affected in a hangover. Now that you know what you're dealing with (and why), it's time to delve into the next area of important discussion. Firstly, let's eliminate some of your questions and concerns. For many of us, hangovers have a sort of cult understanding. We've all probably heard anecdotes and tall-tales of what works and what doesn't. Many times, we're convinced one thing about something, only to later find out that what we believed was completely false. Or, at the very least, not yet supported by science.

Let's explore this area a bit further...

Chapter 4: Live slowly

Waking up slowly, eat breakfast slowly

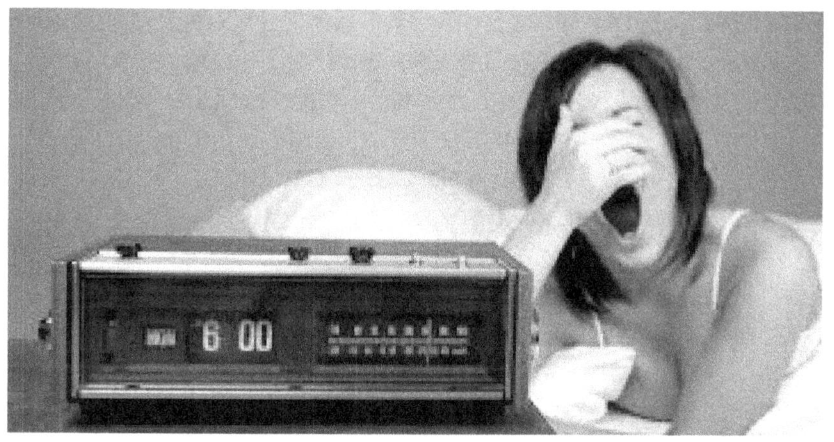

More Precious
Than Gold
What comes to mind when we think about time? Why is it so precious and why do we seek ways to 'make the most of it'?
Let us go back to ancient China in 4,000 BC where the first clocks were invented. In order to demonstrate the idea of time to students, Chinese priests would dangle a rope from the temple ceiling, using knots to represent the hours. They would light it with a flame from the bottom to indicate the passage of time.
Many temples burnt down in those days.
The priests were obviously not too happy about that. So a water bucket method was invented. Holes were

punched in the bottom of a large bucket of water, with markings to represent the hours, and water would flow at a constant rate. The students would measure time by how fast the bucket drained. It was much safer than burning ropes, but more importantly, it taught the students that once time was gone, it could never be recovered.

Of course no one uses water clocks anymore. But the fact that time will eventually run out remains ever true. Time is our most precious possession because, as with the burning rope or water clock, once it is consumed it cannot be replenished. You can always work more hours to earn more money but you cannot do anything to gain more time. Unlike money that can be saved in a bank, or gold that be hidden in a treasure box, time cannot be saved. We have no choice but to spend every moment of it—and every moment that is spent is a moment that is gone forever.

So it seems entirely irrational that we are willing to spend our time making money, but are reluctant to spend our money enjoying our time. We look for the best bargains and think twice before spending money, but often fail to do the same with time. "Wasting" a couple of hours is not as bad as losing a couple of hundred dollars, even though time is far more precious than money. We have the tendency to spend time as if it costs us nothing and this is made worse when you consider that time has an additional "opportunity cost" attached to it. You can divide your money between various things, like clothes, a new car, or a fancy dinner, but when you spend time on a certain activity, you effectively give up the opportunity to spend it on other things. Any benefit that might have been derived, had you chosen to do anything else, would be lost forever.

Time is also priceless because it is truly a miracle that we are here. The odds that we are alive at this moment in time are one in a billion zillion. Think about that. There was only one chance in all the history of this universe that you would have been able to exist, and here you are. If for any reason your father and mother, or any of your grandparents, did not meet at exactly the right time, and at exactly the right place, you would not be here. If any of your ancestors, having gone through wars, famines, and pestilences, did not survive, you would not be here. The odds are astronomically stacked against your existence, but you won the lottery of life. Only you do not know that you won and the prize value in the time given to you is kept hidden. You spend from that credit line without knowing the remaining balance. You realize that whatever you spend cannot be replenished and that lottery of life can only be won once, never twice.

The Value of Time: Work and Leisure

Inventions and technological achievements of the past 100 years were all made for the purpose of providing more leisure time. Cars and planes were invented to make shorten travel. The computer was developed to make work easier. Phones were devised to make communication faster.

Years ago, people thought that in the future there would be nothing to do. The 19th century British economist John Maynard Keynes imagined that in 1930 "our grandchildren would work around three hours a day." In his day, technology had already reduced working hours and so he believed the trend would continue. In fact, according to recent statistics, Americans work 12 hours less each week than they did 40 years ago, and it is even less in Europe.

The main problem for social scientists to tackle seemed to be: what can people do with all that free time? It obviously cannot be placed in a "Time Bank" for future consumption, nor can it be passed on to our children. But free time did not turn out to be a problem after all. Nowadays, people are busier than ever. Time scarcity has increased, especially in the corporate world, and particularly among working parents. It turns out that the problem is less about how much free time we have and more about how we perceive that time. During the Industrial Revolution, when clocks were used to measure labor, the value of time was associated with money. And so the more valuable we perceived our time to be, the less eager we were to "waste it" on leisure, and the scarcer it seemed.

In a recent study carried out at the University of Toronto, two groups of people were asked to listen to the same piece of music, "The Flower Duet" from the opera Lakme. Group A was asked to calculate their hourly wage before the song started, whereas Group B was not asked. The participants in Group A felt less happy, more impatient, and felt that listening to that music was a waste of time. Group B did not. The study showed that most people tend to avoid wasting time so as to maximize the money that they can generate. The additional free time that technology has allowed for is often not spent on enjoying life but rather on working more. And though people may be earning more money, they are not earning more time to spend it in. The higher the paycheck, the scarcer time seems, and the more rushed people become.

Wasted Time?

You have probably heard the saying that money cannot buy happiness. An interesting 2009 Gallup survey, conducted over a period of two years, which gathered 450,000 responses, concluded that people are happier and more satisfied with their lives as their annual income increases. However, when annual income exceeds 75,000 U.S. dollars, life-satisfaction continues to increase but happiness does not. There is an income threshold where money does not contribute to people's emotional well-being.2 This implies that on average, spending time earning more than 75,000 U.S. dollars is not well-spent because it does not make us happier. A central question is therefore this: are we making the most of our limited time?

For now, let us look a little bit further into the "value" of time and "wasted time" as it relates to the culture, country, and the pace of life in the city where we live.

Time & Culture

Our culture affects how we view time, the value we place on time, and how we spend it. Time is perceived differently by Eastern and Western cultures, between countries of the same culture, and even between cities within the same country.

In Western culture, time is viewed as linear. Life is considered a "journey" and death is the "end of the road." The past is behind us and the future is a path that stretches before us. Time is an arrow. There is a beginning and an end to everything. This is based on ideas derived from the Semitic religions (Judaism, Christianity, and Islam), which says that the universe has a clear beginning and will have a clear end on Judgment Day. In those religions, humans are born once and die once.

This linear view of time permeates many facets of Western culture. It explains why Westerners tend to be more focused on the future. It allows them to forecast future events, such as quarterly sales projections, through meticulous planning. You can be extremely confident that the train in Zurich will leave at exactly 10:07 a.m. and arrive at 11:04 a.m. People in these cultures aim to eliminate future unknowns to their best of their abilities. As a result of this linear view, time is considered very precious and limited.

In the linear view, the value of time is equated with money. If you've ever had to deal with an American lawyer or doctor, you would quickly realize that time is money. Americans live in a profit-driven society where time is precious and needs to be utilized as quickly as it is passing. To achieve a decent status in U.S. society, you have to make money, which means you view your time in terms of your hourly wage. There is a linear mathematical relationship between time and money. Equating time and money is also why Americans do not generally tolerate idle time and instead look for ways to save time, such as increasing efficiencies in factory production.

This view is also shared in Britain, Switzerland, Germany, the Netherlands, Austria, and the Scandinavian countries, where time precision for the sake of reducing wasted time is immensely important. Time is extremely regulated for the Swiss, for instance, who made precision their national symbol. Their watches, optical instruments, transportation, and banking industries stand witness to that. Those countries are influenced by the Protestant work ethic, which associates success with working harder and longer hours. Examples of popular idioms are "The early bird catches the worm" and "Never put off to tomorrow what you can do today."

Contrast that with societies that existed in the Soviet Union, where success was achieved by those who made the most by working the least. In Southern European countries, like Italy, Spain, Greece, or the Arab world, success is often associated with privilege, birthright, and connection to authorities. Time is viewed as a rubbery flexible thing, and people are generally not very interested in punctuality or deadlines, and are instead more focused on the end result. A meeting, for instance, is not constrained by clocks but by the discussions themselves, and time can be stretched or manipulated until a reasonable conclusion is met . People from these cultures generally feel less rushed. For them, time runs at a slower pace. While Americans tend to think about time in 5-minute increments, people living in Mediterranean countries and the Middle East do so in 15-minute increments. Popular expressions are: "In Sha' Allah," which in the Arab world means "If God wills," or the Italian proverb, "Since the house is on fire, let us warm ourselves," or the Turkish proverb, "What flares up fast extinguishes soon."

People in Southern European and Middle Eastern countries tend to be more focused on the present, rather than the future, which is likely the reason why these countries are relatively less developed than their northern counterparts. It also explains why people living in Spain, France, and Greece on average save less money, with Italians being the worst savers, as compared to Britain, Netherlands, and Germany, where people tend to be more focused on the future and are among the highest savers in Europe. However, this emphasis on the present is likely why people in Mediterranean cultures appear to enjoy life more, as it is happening now, e.g. the Italian La Dolce Vita (the sweet life), and generally prefer smaller, immediate gratifications over larger, long-term rewards. Now what about the Eastern view on time?

In contrast to the West, time in the East is viewed as cyclical. The sun rises and sets, the seasons follow one another, generations follow generations, governments succeed each other, and this goes on forever. Time is more like a boomerang than an arrow. This idea originates in Eastern religions that believe in reincarnation, like Buddhism, Hinduism, and Taoism. People in cyclical cultures also tend to focus more on the past because they believe they can find links to the present. People's actions in previous lives, known as karma, determines what type of existence they will have after rebirth.

Unlike their West counterparts, Asians are generally not pressed to make quick decisions but instead prefer to contemplate and take their time. For them, time is not scarce; the same opportunities and risks come around again in another cycle, when they are wiser. As a result, they are less disciplined in planning their future and more lenient to go with the flow. Popular idioms are the Chinese proverb, "Wise men are never in a hurry" or the Japanese proverb, "A proposal without patience breaks its own heart."

The Chinese and Japanese, in addition to adopting this hesitant contemplation view of time, differentiate themselves from the rest of the Eastern countries through their keen sense of time. Punctuality is important to them. Chinese often arrive to meetings 15 minutes early, so as to finish on time and maximize efficiency. They appreciate the time that is contributed in a meeting, more than any other Asian countries. But they would still take their time for repeated deliberations before the deal is closed.

The Japanese have a similar deep sense of passing time. This can be observed in how meticulously they are in dividing time. Japanese view time as segmented by tradition. These divisions do not follow Western ideas, where tasks are sequentially allocated to time slots for maximum efficiency, but are more concerned with how much time is given to proper courtesy and tradition. In social gatherings, Japanese have marked beginnings and endings that follow traditional phases. People are expected to conform to the heavily regulated society. This helps in defining where people stand in social and business situations. Exchanging business cards in the first two minutes of a meeting is a clear example that marks the beginning of a relationship. Students in Japanese schools are expected to formally request their teacher to start before the lesson begins. At the end of the class, they offer a ritualistic sign of gratitude. The same rituals apply in tea ceremonies, New Year and midsummer festivities, company picnics, sake-drinking sessions, martial arts sessions, and cherry blossom viewings. These activities are experienced by the Japanese in an unfolding manner. For them, time is segmented into slots defined by tradition, where it is important to do the "right thing at the right time."

The difference between how various cultures view time—as linear, flexible, or cyclic—affects the value people place on time and whether they are more focused on the past, present, or future. Depending on your culture, you either view time as a scarce or abundant.

The Pace of Life

The value of time not only changes with culture, but it also varies between cities of the same country. This is intricately related to the pace of life in any given city.

In an interesting 1990 study, Robert Levine and his colleagues used four indicators to evaluate the pace of life in 36 American cities: the speed with which bank tellers made change, the talking speed of postal clerks, the walking speed of pedestrians, and the proportion of pedestrians wearing wristwatches. Levine found that the Northeastern United States were more fast-paced than the Western United States. Out of the 31 cities surveyed, the three fastest-paced cities were Boston, Buffalo, and New York.3 The three slowest-paced cities were Shreveport, Sacramento, and Los Angeles. They also found that people living in fast-paced cities tend to focus more on making every minute count, which creates more stress. That is why fast-paced cities have higher heart attack death rates and a higher proportion of cigarette smokers.

In 1999, the same researchers carried out another study, which surveyed the largest cities in 31 countries, in an effort to determine what factors contribute to the pace of life. In each country they measured: the pedestrians' walking speed in downtown areas on a clear summer day, the time it took postal workers to complete a standard request for stamps, and they noted the accuracy of the clocks across 15 banks. The results showed that the quick pace of life in cities like Tokyo, London, and Paris causes people to feel rushed and under constant pressure. The United States, Canada, Hong Kong, Taiwan, Singapore, and South Korea fall into the middle group. Slightly below that are the ex-Soviet bloc countries like Hungary, the Czech Republic, Bulgaria, and Romania. The slowest pace of life was found in the relatively non-industrialized countries from Africa (Kenya), Asia (Indonesia), the Middle East (Jordan and Syria), and Latin America (El Salvador, Brazil, and Mexico). Interestingly, the three slowest countries of all were widely associated with a relaxed pace of life. In Brazil, the stereotype of amanha or "tomorrow" means that, whenever it is possible, people will try to put off today's business until tomorrow. In Indonesia, the hour on a clock is often addressed as jam kerat meaning "rubber time." And the slowest of all was Mexico, the characteristic land of la mañana, meaning tomorrow. 4 The researchers also found that the pace of life was slower in hotter cities than cooler ones. This may be due to the fact that in cold cities, natural selection favors people who are more industrious and who keep moving to stay warm. Heat, on the other hand, tends to make people lazier in warmer climates. This could be one of the reasons why northern countries tend to be more economically developed then southern ones.

If we look back at our evolutionary history, we find that, until very recently, time precision was never a critical prerequisite for human survival. In the past, in order to survive, humans needed only to estimate the proper times for eating, sleeping, and working. Nowadays, time is considerably more critical. Aldous Huxley once observed,

To us, the moment 8:17 A.M. means something—something very important, if it happens to be the starting time of our daily train. To our ancestors, such an odd eccentric instant was without significance—did not even exist. In inventing the train, Watt and Stevenson were part inventors of time.

As we saw earlier, when time is viewed as money, hours are measured financially, and people are concerned with how to use time more profitably. As economies grow, time seems scarcer and therefore becomes more valuable. Cities with a higher cost of living raise the price on time. Parisians are more prudent with their time than Mexicans. Pedestrians in Tokyo walk faster than those in Jakarta. In such fast-tempo cities, people earn more money to spend, but do not earn more time to spend it in, making time even more precious. Not having enough time becomes an excuse for not engaging in leisurely experiences, like a relaxing vacation, a quiet dinner, or a concert or theatre performance. As Erich Fromm put it, "Modern man thinks he loses something—time—when he does

not do things quickly. Yet he does not know what to do with the time he gains—except kill it."
Feeling as though one is constantly rushed makes people impatient and impulsive, and affects mental health. In one piece of research from Google, it was found that more than a fifth of internet users will abandon an online video if it takes longer than five seconds to load. The pressure of time can also lead to stress, causing negative health effects such as heart disease, hypertension, headaches, and stomach pain. It can cause chronic anger, depression, bitterness, poor sleep quality, and even a sense of hopelessness. The overall effect of feeling like one has less time is that they are less happy and less satisfied. So what can we do about that? How can we control our perceived speed of time and slow it down to be able to do all the things we want to do?

Slowing time physically is beyond our control. Having a 25-hour day would be great but is not yet possible—although the duration of a day on Earth is getting longer due to our moon's gravity, which acts like a brake and slows down the Earth's spin. As a result, the days are extending by about 1.7 milliseconds each century! But at that rate, you will have to wait 140 million years for one day to finally be 25 hours long! I doubt anyone will be there to see that day, let alone make any use of that extra one hour! (And you might have guessed right, it was far worse for the dinosaurs when the Earth was spinning faster, as they had to fit a full day of work in just 23 hours!)
So, in order to maximize our sense of time, we need to look at how we "experience" time. Drawing on the latest findings in psychology and neuroscience will help us to understand why time seems to pass at different speeds in different situations. We have all

experienced moments in life where time "dragged" or "flew." In situations of extreme fear, you might have experienced moments where time froze. Or you may feel time is speeding up as you grow older. To control the perceived speed of time, we need to understand the factors that create this effect in our minds. Culture and the pace of life are some external factors that influence how limited or abundant time seems. These views can be modified by adjusting the emphasis we put on the past, present, and future and whether our view of time is linear, flexible, or cyclic. But what about the internal factors that affect our time experience? As we go through the book, I will propose a variety of practical tips that will help slow down the pace of time, regardless of which culture or city you live in. With that knowledge, my hope is that you will be able to craft the longest year of your life.

Let us first start with some basics. Our "sense" of time: what is it and how do our brains think about the present, past, and future?

Chapter 5: Good Morning Yoga

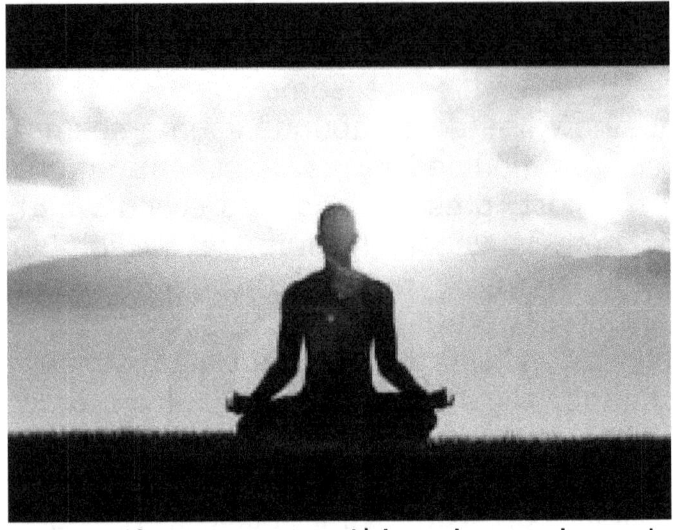

As you practice yoga, nothing is as important as breathing deeply and holding your breath for as long as possible. This is important because holding your breath as you practice whichever asana will ensure you reap the benefits of that specific asana.

Deep/abdominal breathing technique, also called *diaphragmatic breathing,* involves the diaphragm, an important large muscle located between your abdomen and your chest.

When your diaphragm contracts, it moves downward, a movement that leads to the expansion of the abdomen. This process mounts a negative pressure on your chest and forces air into your lungs. This negative pressure helps pull blood into your chest. It also enhances the flow of lymph, known to be rich in immune cells. This causes relaxation of your nervous system and reversal of the stimulation of your parasympathetic nervous system.

Deep breathing is very vital to your overall health and wellbeing. When you engage in yoga and practice deep breathing, you induce a series of physical responses that reverse the changes brought about by stressful, depressive situations. This is how deep/abdominal breathing improves immunity, prevents lung and tissue infections, and induces the relaxation response that leads to less tension and improved general wellbeing.

The calming and reversing effect brought about by deep breathing during yoga happens through the reduction of your heart rate, the tension in your muscles, and by calming your nerves. Since breathing is so important to enjoying the benefits of yoga, it is very important that you learn good breathing techniques. The basics of every deep breathing exercise are to inhale deeply through your nostrils while drawing deeply from your diaphragm/abdomen.

Now that we have established the importance of deep breathing during yoga, let us discuss how to breathe deeply so you can derive the benefits of yoga:

How to Practice Deep/Abdominal Breathing

This type of breathing requires some level of training and mastery before you can get it right. You can follow the steps below to get the best from your deep breathing during yoga exercises:

1. Keep one hand placed on your chest and one on your abdomen. As you inhale through your nostril, the hand on the abdomen ought to rise higher than the one on your chest. This way, you can be sure you are pulling air into the base of your lungs.

2. **As you inhale through your nostrils, visualize the air in the room going into your airways and count from 1-7 while you hold your breath.**

3. Count from 1-8 as you exhale through your mouth. Gently contract your abdominal muscles to ensure any remaining air evacuates your lungs.

4. You can regulate your breath by taking an average of 6 breaths every minute. Repeat this deep/abdominal breathing technique for about 5 times before switching to a different yoga pose.

Having mastered the act of deep/abdominal breathing, let us now look at how, by using different yoga poses, you can achieve different ends such as boosting immunity, building stamina, and fighting stress and anxiety.

Before we do that, however, let us lay some ground rules for your yoga practice.

Chapter 6: The Hidden Influences That Shape you are Eating Habits

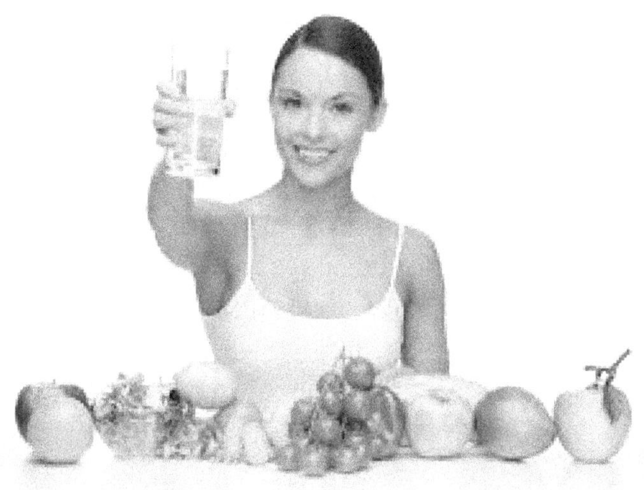

- Healthy eating enables your mind, to link itself to body and soul. Your body will begin valuing the adjustment in your diet and you will feel greatly improved. Healthy eating is truly the healthiest approach to shed pounds. And, a healthy nutritional low-calorie diet and an activity regimen, help control maladies and ageing.

- Realize that the reason we tend to begin putting on weight is that we devour a larger number of calories than the measure of calories that we consume. And, mot of us have battled with our eating habits in light of an assortment of elements. The amount and nature of the great unhealthy foods that we consume are the things that make us unhealthy. Couple both of these variables to a bustling work routine, and it turns out to be exceptionally hard to eat a healthy diet. We have to make healthy eating a need in our lives. So we should begin a regimen.

- Begin by getting yourself a new food chart which is in the shape of a pyramid. Make this your manual for starting to eat healthy. Initially, recognize the food classes and the amounts that can be eaten. Realize which organic product, vegetables, seafood, and meats are prescribed.

- When you do your grocery shopping, take a stab at getting the freshest foods grown in the ground, and if possible purchase natural creations. Endeavor to eliminate with soda pops and junk food from your grocery list. This is the principal issue that we have in the country. It is anything but difficult to pull up to a fast-food drive-through and get a fast meal.

Breakfast

- Breakfast is the most critical meal of the day. You have to begin your day with a nutritious meal. Your breakfast meal ought to incorporate organic products or natural product juices, oats (low in sugar), low-fat grains and eggs. Endeavor to be light on the bacon, yet If it's an unquestionable requirement, recall that you need to keep your cholesterol in check. If you don't have enough time in the morning to make yourself a healthy meal, have a breakfast bar. There are a lots of them available that are nutritious and low in calories.

Lunch

- With regards to lunchtime abstain from eating fast foods. Make your own lunch or eat a salad with chicken from the market or at an eatery. You can eat out at eateries but be aware of what you are eating and the dangers of the parts that you eat. You'd be amazed how in one meal you can consume all the calories that you ought to consume in the whole day.

Dinner

- Attempt to have your dinner at an early hour at night or late evening. This is one of the greatest mix-ups many individuals commit. They have dinner late at night and nod off in the blink of an eye a while later. If you have a healthy dinner early and get eager to eat later at night, simply have a low-calorie snack and water.

Top Tips for Healthy eating Meals

- Figure out how to plan healthy meals. You ought to set up your meals low in salt and fat. Have a go at broiling your meats as opposed to browning, and abstain from utilizing a lot of sugar and salt in the recipes. There are a lot of seasonings that improve the taste of your foods while keeping them healthy and low in calories.

- Drink no less than eight glasses of water a day. This will enable your digestive system to consume calories and take out poisons from your body. In addition, drinking water encourages you with your stomach related framework. Be careful with drinking excessively squeezed juices. In spite of the fact that juices are healthy, they are as often as possible high in sugar and in calories.

- Fill your icebox and washroom with healthy foods and dispose of the greater part of the junk food. If you have junk food at home you will presumably, in the long run, eat it. An ideal approach to keep to a healthy diet is to just have healthy food in your home. There are a lot of healthy snacks accessible to purchase.

- When feasting at an eatery keep up your teaching. Avoid the bread basket or advise the server to expel it from the table. There are numerous eateries that offer a choice of healthy meals; some even give the meal's calories and nutritional data on the menu.

- Once your eating habits change at home you will find that it is substantially simpler to keep to your healthy habits when you are eating out. Low in salt, low in sugar, and no broiling ought to be your primary concerns while setting up your meals. Segment control is the other.

- Try not to avoid a meal. Skipping meals is not healthy. Your body goes into starvation mode and this backs off your digestion. If you are endeavoring to get more fit, skipping meals will defeat your endeavors. Three meals per day and a few snacks is the healthier approach. A few specialists even suggest five small meals every day.

- When you have executed a healthy eating regimen you will find that you will lose the urge to eat fast food or junk food. The desire that you once had for cheeseburgers and French fries is no longer there. Your days of experiencing that drive-through are finished.

- It is imperative to restrain your intake of alcohol. Drinking alcohol reduces your digestion, as well as having calories that you are drinking. Attempt to quit drinking or restrict it to only two or three beverages at the end of the week. If you're a beer consumer, drink light beer or have a go at switching to red wine, which is healthier.

- Finally, adhere to your objective of healthy eating foods. If you have been eating unhealthy for a considerable length of time it could be a troublesome change; however, If you take the time and follow the tips given here you ought to be well on your way to eating in a healthy way.

Every restorative investigation has demonstrated the constructive outcomes a healthy diet can have. It can enable you to control diabetes, bring down your cholesterol level, bring down your hazard for coronary illness, help with weight issues, and more. Eating a healthy diet additionally, assists with resting issue and keeps your mind more engaged. Begin healthy eating

Chapter 7: Design Your Day: Be More Productive, Set Better Goals

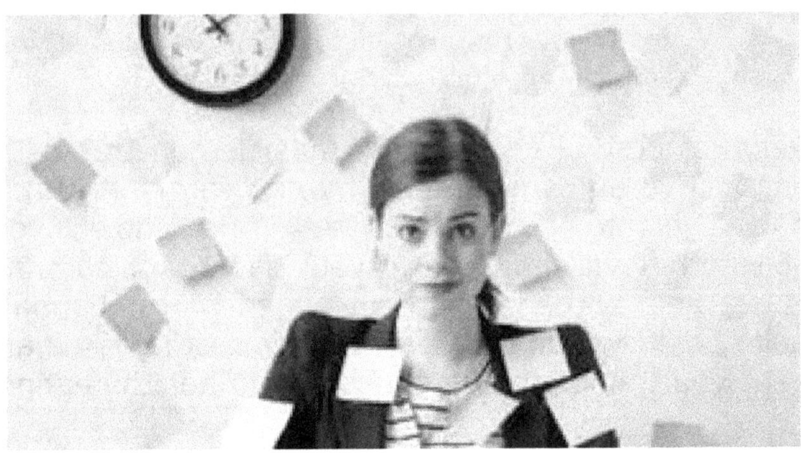

Now that we looked at the various reasons behind a person's habit of procrastinating, let us look at some of the things that you can do immediately to fix yours. But remember, these will only be effective if you practice it regularly and not take it up on a trial basis. You must be persistent and consistent, and only then will you be able to see positive results.

Make a to-do list

The first step for you to adopt is to make a "to-do" list. As simplistic and old fashioned as it sounds, it is one of the best ways for you to start on your mission. Write it down on a piece of paper in the traditional way, as opposed to jotting it down on your cell phone.

When you write it down, you feel more connected with it and be more dedicated to pursuing it.

The main purpose of writing things down is for you to have a visual reminder of the tasks that you must be doing instead of sitting around and wasting time. Once you start to do this task with dedication, your mind will stop needing a physical list. It will begin to make a mental "to-do" list and you will start ticking one off, with much ease.

Go for the tough tasks first

After you make the list, you must give them appropriate ranks. These ranks will be based on the level of difficulty with the toughest task placed at top. When you start performing these tasks, you must go for the toughest one first and do the easiest one last.

The logic behind this theory is that, when posed with a set of tasks which range from easy to difficult, 90% of people will opt for the easy one, and when it comes to the tough one, they will avoid it and think of doing it at a later time. So, it is best to go for the tough tasks first and then tackle the easy ones.

De-clutter

The next step involves you de –cluttering your space. If you live in a house where there is a lot of clutter scattered around or have a cluttered office space where there are a lot of files and papers strewn, then you are bound to feel lazy. And when you feel lazy, you will not feel like doing anything. You will keep delaying it, and it will continue on until and unless you clear your space and get organized.

You must invest in some organizing baskets and racks that will help you keep your house and office clean and try to dispose items that you don't need. With a clutter free environment, you will also help safeguard your health and not promote stress or depression, which can be causes for procrastination.

Time your tasks

Before you start with your tasks, you must attach a deadline to each one. If you go about a task without a time frame in mind, then you will end up spending too much time doing just one thing and have none left for the rest.

When you make the "to –do" list, you can also jot down the time within which you wish to finish the task. You must try your best to finish it within that time frame. If you are not sure how much time it will take, then perform the task once and write down an inner and upper limit depending on it. Ideally, the time you set must be slightly lesser than the time that you took to finish it the first time.

Do not multi task

When you start performing the tasks, you must not do too many at the same time. If you do, you will start to tire out faster. Your limbic system will start pushing in the notion of procrastination and force you to delay the task.

So, when you wish to do something, then concentrate only on one thing and not worry or consider anything else. And if you feel that you are taking too much time on one task and you should have finished by now, then speed up the task and try to finish it within the next 10 to 15 minutes. If it does not happen, then move to the next task immediately. With time, you will understand the value of time and not have to move on abruptly.

Tackle distractions

You must tackle all distractions. In your day to day life, there will be just so many that you will start to lose count after a certain point in time. You must have a fool proof plan to keep these distractions at bay. You must make up your mind to concentrate on nothing but the task at hand, even if there is a clear and apparent distraction.

You must tell yourself that you will deal with the distraction only after you are done with the task and not during or in between. These distractions can be people, passions, pets, or any such, which might prevent you from giving your task 100%.

Be reasonable

Always be reasonable in your approach to your tasks. When you set out to correct your problem of procrastination, do not hope to do it within a few days or weeks. Remember that you are battling against a force that is quite strong and quite old, and the only way you can beat it is through patience and persistence.

The time that it will take you to change a habit will depend on your capacity to change and how long it generally takes for you to adopt or change a habit. You might take lesser time, if you put in more than your 100% into it.

At the same time, do not try to make everything perfect. Perfection is not possible in all fields of life, and if you try too hard to be perfect, then you will end up discouraging yourself. Always aim to give it your best and forget the rest.

Keep motivated

You must keep yourself motivated at all times. You must have a book to record your progress, which will allow you to understand if you are headed in the right direction. You must never give up and keep at it until you know for sure that you are changing.

Remember, you must do this for yourself, and for your own good, and only because you want to kick the habit and get faster results. If you are doing it under influence or under someone's instructions, then it will not work for you.

You might feel overwhelmed at times. During such times, you must tell yourself that this is for your own good and forge ahead.

Reinforcement

When it comes to using reinforcement to foster your growth, you must be able to implement both positive and negative reinforcement. When it comes to positive reinforcement, you must be able to reward yourself from time to time. And this reward must only come through if you feel that you have made enough and comprehensible progress.

You must be able to measure the progress and understand that you are not procrastinating tasks any more or at least to the extent that you once used to. The reward can be anything like a nice meal at a fancy restaurant or something material, like a shoe or dress you always wanted to own. The value of the reward must be in proportion to the progress. So, if your progress was big, then so should the reward, and if it was small, then so should the reward.

Negative reinforcement should be the opposite. If you feel that you are not making any progress and still procrastinate as usual, then you must try and deny yourself a certain thing that you are fond of. It can be an item of food like chocolates or even a perfume that you love.

Once you use it as a prize, you will be motivated to keep going and win the item back. You will work harder, and once you know that you have made progress, you can reward yourself with the item that you withheld.

Find a partner

The last step is for you to find a partner. When you practice the above steps with someone else, who is also interested in kicking their habit of procrastination, then you will keep yourself better motivated.

You will be able to assess your progress better and also know where you are going wrong. You will know where to make amends depending on looking at the other person's mistakes. You can hold regular assessment tests and rate each other's progress, which will help both of you.

Chapter 8: Purpose Driven Life divide into small targets

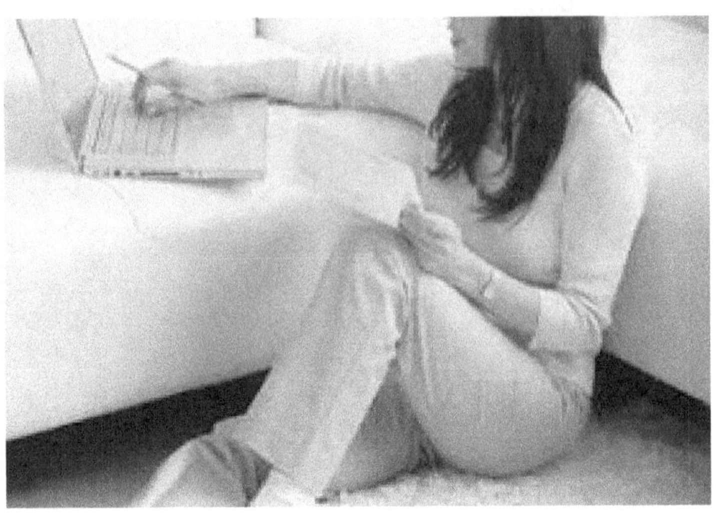

One of the most common questions I get asked by clients is "What is my life purpose?" or "What am I here to do?" I know that many of you are plagued by this question. Or even if you have a pretty good understanding of what your life purpose is, you probably still need guidance on what steps to take in order to fulfill it more effectively and abundantly. In keeping with our theme of aligning with your life purpose in January I thought I would share some practical, simple steps you can take to fulfilling your life purpose.

1. Decide what it is you truly want. A soul moves by desire. In order to discover what you are here to do, take a look within at your innermost desires. Ask yourself, what do I want? Is that what I really want? What else do I want? The deeper you can go with this process, the stronger it will be for you. Be sure to

discern if it is something that you REALLY want, or whether it is something you think you should do, or someone else wants you to do. I recently helped my client Megan work through this process of deciding what she really wanted. She had been talking about moving back to her home state of New York to be close to her family for quite some time. So when I asked her to write a list of the things that she really, really wanted, a move back to New York was at the top of her list. As we worked on this goal for her, I kept coming up against resistance and her reasons why a move to New York would be difficult. For example, for financial reasons, her husband might not get a job and doesn't like commuting to the city, she couldn't afford the same size house in NY as she has in VA, etc.It is normal to have to work through limiting beliefs in order to have what you desire. But this was different. It really seemed like there was no positive solution. She wanted her sister and her Mom to move back to NY from VA also, and she felt she had to pay for them too because they couldn't afford it. She believed this was the only way for the family to be together because, "My other sister will never move from NY."I realized that her motive for everyone to be together was coming from a sense of responsibility to look after everyone else. I helped her to see that she can't interfere with her sister's free will not to move from NY. Sometimes, what we want is not the same as what others want and so we have to accept their choices and let it go. Finally I asked her, "Is this really want you want?" She realized her answer was "no." I asked her how that felt. She shared with me that it felt like a big sense of relief. Once she had let go of that desire that was really authentic for her to move states, she could freely work on her other goals to open a yoga studio and build an extension on her house, without the burden of thinking she should hold back from doing anything new 'cause she might be moving soon. What a relief! Are you desires really authentic to you? Or are they coming from unclear motives, like Megan's sense of responsibility to look after her family? Be sure that you are clear within.

2. You have no limitations. I can't tell you the number of times people have told me, "I don't know what my life purpose is. I don't know what I want." Then five minutes later end up sharing a secret desire they have for a new career or business or hobby. It's probably not that you don't know what you want. It' s more likely that you are placing limiting beliefs on yourself so you don't believe that you can do it. You automatically decide, "That can't be right, that's not my life purpose." I worked with a client recently who told me she was looking for her life purpose. She said she had always wanted to be a healer but didn't know what her life purpose was. As simple as it sounds, I confirmed for her that her life purpose is to be a healer. We worked through all the limiting beliefs she was holding. For example, that it was not practical, she would never earn any money doing that, she was too old, etc. The only thing stopping her from being a successful healer is the negative beliefs she is holding about it. She is creating her own reality. When you think about what you really want, how quickly are you to dismiss it as being too scary or too impractical? Just for once, try believing that you really can do this. It's incredible how quickly things will change. I have lived in this house for 9 years not believing I could ever afford to renovate the basement. Three months ago during the Angelic Business Secrets class I taught, I declared that I was going to set a bold money goal to create the money to renovate my basement. Now the

work is underway! The shift can be so easy when you just believe differently, more positively about your life. 3. Set and Declare your Intentions! My friend Cynthia reminded me of the importance of setting your intentions when I got together with her this past weekend. When she had her baby last year, she only had 6 weeks of paid leave available to her. She knew she really needed & wanted to be home with her baby for 3 months. She declared that "It's all going to work out" and just stopped worrying about it - even though a part of her mind was thinking she was crazy! She let it go and trusted that the solutions would appear. During the time she was on maternity leave, she was able to sell her car, and got a tax refund that kept the income that she needed to support her and her son perfectly. When it was time to go back to work, she was concerned about finding a great childcare provider that she trusted. She set the intention to find a childcare provider who she would trust just like her mom. She discovered a daycare center down the street who even has the same name as her mom. The teachers there are like second mothers to her son and she couldn't be happier with the arrangements. The key when you set your intention is to let go of the "How." If you worry and fret about what is going to happen or how you are going to do it, your intellectual nature will start worrying and getting scared. You'll do more harm than good! Set your intention. Declare it to another person to make it even more powerful. (It helped me to declare my basement renovation intention publicly to my group of 21 participants in the Angelic Business Secrets course! It kept me accountable!)Then, stay relaxed and open to noticing the opportunities when they come up. Do your research. Find what's out there. Use your intuition and your inner guidance to discern when action needs to be taken. Follow through! When it feels right, do it!

4. Set clear and specific goals. Another reason that many people stay stuck wondering what they are supposed to be doing with their lives, is that they are very vague with their direction. They kind of have an idea of what they want, or don't even think about it because their day-to-day life takes over. If you want your life to change, you must take the time to be clear and specific about what your goals are. Don't be afraid of the word "goals." A goal is a signpost along the road that gives you direction. It gives you a road map and a guide for what actions to take now in order to reach that signpost. The more clear and specific you can be, the quicker you will reach your goal. This is because your energy will be aligned with it, and your angels will move in to help you more because they are clear on your intentions too. If you are indecisive and wishy-washy, you make it difficult for your angels to help you manifest. They don't know what direction you are going in! When Richard and I decided to renovate our basement, we had a contractor come over and give us an estimate on the cost to finish the walls and ceiling. We had our number. That became the financial goal to work towards and has given us extra motivation and drive to create the money and save it aside. It is easier to manifest money when that money has a purpose. It is more difficult to manifest money just for money's sake. Decide what you want, get the facts on the cost, the time involved and what needs to be done. Write your plan and set to work with your magical intentions to allow it to happen creatively! Be flexible along the way. Enjoy creating a magical year in 2013 aligned with your life purpose!